Born and raised in Chesterfield, his life was shaped dramatically after he was diagnosed with Bipolar Affective Disorder having spent a stressful time in France working to learn French. Having been sectioned and spent several months recovering, he was motivated to write about his own mental health issues, how others can recover, and how recovery can help patients, staff and all stakeholders to evolve given how much pressure there is facing our health services.

to Ben

hope you enjoy reading it

Much Love

Andrew

Andrew Spriggs

The Recovery Model: The Truth of Its Value

Austin Macauley Publishers™
London • Cambridge • New York • Sharjah

A CIP catalogue record for this title is available from the British Library.

ISBN 9781398492646 (Paperback)
ISBN 9781398492653 (ePub e-book)

www.austinmacauley.com

First Published 2023
Austin Macauley Publishers Ltd®
1 Canada Square
Canary Wharf
London
E14 5AA

I would like to most sincerely thank the following people and organisations:

Dr Julie Repper – ImRoc.

Mr Dave Riley – NHS Merseycare.

Mr Jeremy Coutinho – South West London and St Georges Mental Health Trust.

(all for their help and cooperation in writing this book)

Camden and Islington NHS Foundation Trust for their assistance.

Mr Ifti Majid – Chief Executive at Derbyshire Healthcare NHS Foundation Trust (for his immense interest and support for the relevance of the book for the work his staff do).

Mrs Lisa Rowbottom – CPN at Derbyshire Healthcare NHS Foundation Trust – for her constant support for my mental health and interest in this book.

Dr Paul Rowlands – Consultant Psychiatrist at Derbyshire Healthcare NHS Foundation Trust – for his great interest and support for my mental health and this book.

It comes as no surprise to me the pressures the NHS faces, budget cuts forcing fewer staff to cover greater work-loads. Coronavirus has in itself added a new dimension with staff having to work remotely, service users are unable to see their key workers and fewer members of staff manning NHS premises. Getting back to pre-COVID levels of service is challenging enough but what does the long-term future look like given the way we are operating?

How can we progress the NHS as the UK's largest employer if we do not strip down and look at what our core issues are? Why are there staff shortages? Why do we keep needing more staff? Why are budgets so stretched?

Our nurses, doctors, support workers, occupational therapists and administrative staff amongst many others deserve to go to work supported with the knowledge that they will not be expected to make decisions that are out of their remit. They deserve to have support when things get stressful and to have their voices heard and, where possible, their views taken on board. How can this happen in a more naturally progressive way? It is my view that changes from a 'bottom-up' angle would not only benefit those receiving care but would greatly reduce pressures felt by staff working within mental health services. We need to help those most who fall through the net, who are in need of more help than what is currently on offer so those in charge of our care can work on a broader scale to offer more assistance.

"For many people experiencing mental health challenges, the concept of recovery is about staying in control of their life despite experiencing a mental health problem.

"(Leamy et al, 2011) Deegan (1996, p.97) defines recovery as: "…re-establish(ing) a new and valued sense of integrity and purpose within and beyond the limits of the disability; the aspiration is to live, work and love in a community in which one makes a significant contribution…" (Maybery, D and Reupert, A)

In using a strengths-based solution-focused approach the basic building blocks of good recovery practice are taken as being fundamental:

- ***Belief that recovery is a possibility***
- ***Respect***
- ***Encouragement***
- ***Optimism***
- ***Empathy***
- ***Anti-oppressive practice***
- ***Self-awareness and reflective practice***
- ***Understanding the principles of recovery***
- ***Clear boundaries***
- ***Accepting the person's definition of the problem***
- ***Objectifying and not personalising the person's behaviour.***

Everyone is accountable for their actions; the answer lies in looking at how we can help ourselves and be helped and in doing so also assist our health-care professionals so they can help those coming into the service in crisis. How are we helping those who help those in need? By revisiting how we help individuals in the first place, we can identify how many slip through the net, as well as critically assessing how we help those in need, we can look at individual case studies so we know how we can improve things for everybody.

This book will look at a range of components that formulate the recovery model and show how individual recovery can greatly help not only the patients themselves but all stakeholders in different ways; making it a widely beneficial strategy.

The Importance of Meaningful Work, Hobbies and Recreational Activities

Being in suitable work provides a structure that helps people to feel valued and gives a purpose to each day. Some patients can find work that suits them which is full-time, 9–5pm or part-time. Others may try various jobs or may have been in a career that previously exacerbated their mental health. Some may have found work anxiety provoking, others feel the pressure more than other workers, which results in time off work and low mood. For many, the politics within the workplace can be the dominant stressor.

Finding that balance in terms of suitable work and work which is perhaps somewhat ambitious is a journey we all go on. For mental health sufferers, the balance can be much finer:

a few too many hours and it can upset the mood, too much time on their hands can be a major source of stress and depression. Many are capable of permanent work; others prefer temporary ongoing work or project work. Being in work can feel at times like a life sentence, however; particularly when there is no 'end' to the job, full-time work can take its toll. All workplaces are sources of stress at any one time. The problem becomes acute when there are multiple sources of stress. This can really upset the 'applecart'.

It does take time to adjust to work after lengthy periods off work. However, it can often be a case of trial and error or trial and improvement. Why is it important to find that balance? Well, being stressed is no fun and for those with long-term mental health conditions it is not sustainable. Too much stress can cause emotional distress and can upset the chemical imbalance and then mood. It can take changes in medication to resolve matters caused by stress, aside from any emotional and psychological interferences.

Finding a supportive workplace and suitable job raises self-esteem, improves confidence and provides motivation to complete other tasks. Often jobs may arise relating to a patient's hobby or personal interests, aligned with their core values. When job responsibilities conflict with their personal values, there is a likelihood that that person will disadvantage themselves because the particular responsibility goes against their core beliefs. This can cause huge amounts of stress that build up over a relatively short period of time. Indeed, the Royal College of Psychiatrists provides the following justification for those with health conditions who are considering work as their next step:

Work as a social and health benefit

- *Provides a monetary reward – but also non-financial gains, including social identity and status, social contacts and support, a means of structuring and occupying time, it provides activity and involvement and a sense of personal achievement*
- *Enhances quality of life*
- *Promotes social inclusion, linking the individual to society*
- *Unemployment is linked with premature death, development of mental health problems, increased use of mental health services, increased risk of suicide*

Work as a rights issue

- *Article 23 of the United Nations Declaration of Human Rights: "Everyone has a right to work, to free choice of employment, to just and favourable conditions of work and to protection against unemployment."*
- *Valuing people with disabilities includes promoting respect, self-determination and empowerment*
- *Prejudice and discrimination is a major obstacle to people with mental health problems gaining work*

Work as an economic issue

- *A large proportion of public money is spent on welfare benefits for the unemployed and almost 25% of invalidity payments are paid to people with mental health problems*
- *Further costs to society come in the form of loss of productivity due to absenteeism and presenteeism*

Having interests are crucial too. Thespian lovers claim that acting and singing are the best way to switch off from any underlying stressors, as you can switch off automatically from day-to-day issues while gym lovers say 30 minutes on the treadmill cannot be beaten in terms of effectiveness at relieving stress. Exercise also raises the mood and improves self-esteem, as well as working off the Sunday lunch or afternoon tea! Being able to access the gym when things start to become unstuck can really help to put things back in perspective and reduce the length of low mood spells. Creative writing and drawing can offer therapy from stress and trauma, as well as writing a book. Gardening can be a great tension relief – when full of negativity the work acts as a therapeutic release.

It is also important to balance all work and interests with down time to watch a film or listen to music or meditate. Having a mental health condition means having a more finely-tuned balance to those who do not suffer mental illness. This section is the first segment to be discussed which contributes to a patient's quality of living and can be partly or wholly incorporated into a person's education via a peer-support training class or training programme.

Financial Help for Those with Mental Health Diagnoses

Having a mental health condition makes you more likely to be financially vulnerable. When mood is elevated it can be easy to spend more money and accrue debts. Also, budgeting and doing income and expenditure forms are harder to do in these circumstances. While it is important to recognise that mental illness affects up to one in three of us, there are plenty of rich and famous individuals who have suffered mental hardship as a result of debt crises. In fact, for those who appear rich and famous they can actually have underlying spiralling debts totalling hundreds of thousands of pounds when they live beyond their means. Debt caused by mental ill health or as a contributor of such does not discriminate.

On a limited income through work, it is always best to make enquiries as to what benefits are available and advice on budgeting is available at Citizens Advice or your bank. Benefit forms can be complex so it is best to ask advice from your Community Psychiatric Nurse, Citizens Advice or Welfare Rights. Benefits are there for people who are more likely to struggle due to a health condition and may need more time off work. This is not wasted money but the Government's support to aid recovery.

Debts are also a very contentious issue and it is very easy to bury your head in the sand and try to avoid the issue. I accrued thousands of pounds of debt from my previous book-publishing packages. I was paying just enough to keep myself afloat, yet still spending on my credit cards. This was fine while I was in work until I had to leave on ill-health grounds. Facing my debts was scary and distressing, yet with support from my nurse and StepChange, a leading debt charity, I arranged a plan to start paying it back. Debts are something that can easily get out of control, so it's never a bad time to ask for help.

StepChange explain the difficulties that those who are mentally vulnerable encounter with debt and they include some interesting facts:

"In 2017, one in five of our clients had an additional vulnerability (such as illness) on top of their problem debt. Our new research shows that they tend to be in a notably worse financial position than other clients.

"This underpins the importance of the financial sector's current focus on vulnerability and cements our view that better safety nets are needed to prevent vulnerable people from suffering disproportionate difficulty.

"There are many reasons for vulnerability according to the new analysis in Breaking the Link: a closer look at vulnerable people in debt. Among our vulnerable clients, the overwhelmingly most common reason was mental health difficulty (43%), followed by physical disability (4.7%), cancer (4.6%) and poor health (4.1%).

"Debt problems are closely associated with certain forms of vulnerability, especially illness. 77% of clients with a terminal illness and 68% of clients with cancer, cited illness as the main cause of their debt problems. Among those with mental health issues, 40% said illness was the main reason for their debt. Two in five vulnerable clients overall said that the main reason for them falling into debt was illness.

"However, vulnerability can derive from situations, as well as personal characteristics – bereavement, relationship

breakdown, poor treatment by firms and many other features could all make someone vulnerable at certain times, even if the vulnerability is temporary.

"Vulnerable clients were significantly more likely than other clients to have a net household income of under £10,000, and significantly less likely to have a net household income over £20,000. 45% of vulnerable clients had a deficit budget (with less money coming in than going out), even after budgeting advice, compared with 30% of clients as a whole.

"Over two thirds of vulnerable clients were receiving benefits, compared with half of those clients without a vulnerability. Yet their benefits were less likely to prevent them facing a budget shortfall, with 40% facing a deficit budget compared with 37% of clients without a vulnerability in receipt of benefits.

"Vulnerable clients were more likely than other clients to be in arrears on household bills such as rent, utilities or council tax. And they spent an average of 70% of their income on essential household bills and food compared with 65% among other clients.

"Commenting on the findings, StepChange Debt Charity chief executive Phil Andrew said: "Among our clients, those who are vulnerable typically show higher levels of financial distress – but that shouldn't be inevitable. While there has been progress, it's clear that the finance sector, regulators and the debt advice sector could all still do more to help break the link between being vulnerable and being significantly worse off."

Facing debt is the first step and is challenging but through recovery peer support it can be easier to face up to these acute problems and move forwards each other's recovery journey. By hearing other's accounts, it can provide hope and belief that these issues can and will be overcome. It is the most daunting step but once a repayment plan has been started, there is a certain level of satisfaction at seeing the debt shrink. If you are eligible for financial support, often recovery classes provide the gateway to finding out more information about what you may be entitled to, being a great support to help see you through any difficult times if work has caused the issue or there are other external issues.

Establishing And Maintaining Good Relationships

A supportive network is essential to maintaining good mental health and one which can be explored in a recovery peer-support setting. Many who attend such groups do not have any other local connections and may be struggling emotionally or they may have 'toxic' relationships that drag them down and, as such, they find these very difficult to break free from. Good and better relationships can be explored, so the patient can find out more amongst others and the peer-support worker. For example, they may be able to access support from other groups by word of mouth and also make new friends and contacts there so they start to feel more integrated. Those who offer information in these groups may feel happy to help and this may, in fact, boost their confidence – helping a peer in more need.

Indeed, a study carried out by Harvard University highlighted the importance of social connections and interaction following a vast research project:

"In 1938, Harvard University began following 724 participants as part of the longest-running study on human development in history. The study was developed to determine what makes us happy. The study explored every part of who we are, from physical and psychological traits to social life and IQ to learn how we can flourish. Findings from the study were published in the 2012 book "Triumphs of Experience", with key results showing that happiness and health aren't a result of wealth, fame or working hard but come instead from our relationships:

- ***Social connections are really good for us and loneliness kills. People who are more socially connected to family, friends or community are happier, physically healthier and live longer than people who are less well connected.***
- ***It's not just the number of friends you have and it's not whether or not you're in a committed relationship but it's the quality of your close relationships that matters. Living in conflict or within a toxic relationship is more damaging than being alone.***
- ***Good relationships don't just protect our bodies, they protect our brains. Good quality relationships were related to sharper memory."***

'No Force First' And 'Integrated Supported Housing Schemes'

Recovery strategies have been used largely to empower individuals and service users from needing further excessive care. Recovery is something which we are all in, whether in hospital or out in the community. It is non-discriminate, non-judgemental and can freely impact positively on us all. It is a bottom-up approach whereby decisions about helping those in need are made by those down below. It is essentially about learning lessons and overcoming obstacles that confront us in our daily lives.

While this approach looks at how using the recovery model can help service users in need and the benefits to staffing, there is also growing evidence as to how the use of recovery strategies can save NHS Trusts a lot of money. It is evident that some Mental Health Trusts have had great success at developing recovery strategies that have been not only financially viable but also practically and emotionally suitable for all concerned.

A report entitled *Recovery: The Business Case* by ImROC (2017) has found economic evidence that providing training on using no force within in-patient settings, as per "No Force First" (which NHS Mersey Care initiated), has huge benefits for all stakeholders, including patients, staff and management. Indeed, this initiative looked at viewing the narrative from 'containment' to 'recovery'. In essence, it is about eliminating and reducing the need for restraint of patients on in-patient wards, and also about removing blanket rules as such and focusing on individual needs, therefore enabling a listening culture. If service users feel there are barriers between themselves and staff in general, or certain members of staff, this could be a potential catalyst for tension.

When I was sectioned after trying to leave, there was somewhat of a barrier between myself and the staff to the extent that the staff seemed to be working against me. Being restrained is not only incredibly traumatic but demoralising and once dosed up on PM medication strips the last few bits of confidence away. Contrary to the care I received at times, being calm towards service users in distress is critical for their ongoing well-being. Those in authority are usually able to and should usually be able to diffuse difficult distressing situations. Talking to someone with a raised voice is more likely to see a continuation of tension, seeing the service user as a mental health problem. Exploring why the service user has behaved in a certain way can de-escalate the issue so that it does not become a problem again. Once understood and listened to calmly, the service user feels their voice has been heard.

'No Force First' at NHS Mersey Care was evaluated and the findings were incredibly positive. The year to August 2017 saw a 23% reduction on assaults to staff. In 2012/13 NHS Mersey Care was 8% above the national average for assaults on staff; in 2015/16 the figure had dropped to 65% below the national average. Indeed, not only are the wards safer but in the year to August 2017 the Trust saved £249,069 in staff sickness absence costs. However, most importantly, as a result of these changes it has been widely reported as positive feedback that staff feel safer as a result of 'No Force First'.

It is also important to remember those 'mental health problems' that are maybe sitting smoking or gazing at the wall, wondering what to do with themselves. You know those on a section 2 or section 3, who look like they're institutionalised staring at the wall?! I was very lucky to have a family to support me when I left hospital but what do some other patients have? Do they have any interests that could be used to empower them? How are they going to manage leaving hospital? What are their short-term and long-term solutions? How can you find ways to empower patients, enabling them to live better, healthier lives? Are patients behaving in a challenging manner as a result of their previous traumas? What about handovers, are they objective, positive and recovery-focused? How can you involve these ones in activities that strengthen their understanding as to why they are in hospital and also prepare them for life after hospital?

Providing in-patients with activities or the ability to try different activities can help them to focus on a routine in what is a very strange setting. Regular appointments for classes or one-to-one appointments can really help the individual to identify what led him or her to admission and how they can learn from their experiences. This frequently occurs but this book is more about dotting the i's and crossing the t's. Such amazing work has already been done and is being done. But can we do more?

The answer is yes, more can always be done. A further study, which was researched and outlined in *Recovery: The Business Case* (2017) by ImROC, looked at Camden and Islington NHS Foundation Trust in London where they created an 'Integrated supported housing scheme' with 15 self-contained flats for patients with complex mental health needs. They created specific safety features that enable risk to be managed whilst being able to hold group sessions or workshops in shared communal areas. Camden and Islington

NHS Foundation Trust provide on-site support and help customers to avoid eviction. The Trust has managed to reduce hospital admissions and costs in excess of £440,000 per annum and has saved £900,000 overall since opening. The two years prior to the scheme saw 408 weeks of hospital admissions; the two years afterwards saw this dramatically reduce to 57.7 weeks. Since opening in 2012 the scheme has enabled the Trust to free up hospital beds by means of a large reduction in admissions and provide patients with better health and a more positive outlook, as well as building their confidence and improving the life skills that are needed.

So, why have I mentioned the strategies that the aforementioned Trusts have taken? Partly because I was sectioned when I was 20 and it was the most frightening experience of my life, being restrained and injected with tranquillisers. Really, the most frightening experience of my life. But I also believe that there is, as stated above, evidence which suggests that using alternative methods to avoid forced restraint can help both patient and staff member and, ultimately, save a lot of money. Empowering the vulnerable gives them confidence and reassurance that they can pull out all the stops to recover and stay on the right path. Many are not so fortunate as I was to have my family to fall back on and support me. Giving purpose and hope to everyone's personal needs or interests and adapting these to fit in with their recovery plan could assist in eliminating any need for restraint and help the individual adapt to life after admission. The flats provide a solution to prevent readmission. Reflecting on those who were also in my ward, the flats could have helped some of them to readjust gradually to 'normal' life.

Recovery Colleges

Once in the community, encouraging patients to attend a recovery college can greatly improve their chances of staying well. Having a WRAP plan, a 'Wellness Recovery Action Plan', which could be included as part of a recovery class session, can greatly help those in need to know what helps them best when they are in crisis. Attending classes is something that many may benefit from on an educational level, as well as health and psychological input, if they have been discharged and need support and may not have been able to be supported by family or friends.

As stated in my previous book, *Mental Health Recovery: Protecting our Front Line NHS Staff*, attending such classes has proven successful in reducing hospital readmissions. It gives structure to the individual's life by looking at what triggers mental illness and how they can take responsibility to make changes. It is also an opportunity for service users to mix with others and forms a basis for how they can proceed with their lives. There is, as previously stated, significant evidence to suggest that an individual with mental health needs who attends classes following a hospital admission is less likely to need to be readmitted.

South West London and St George's Mental Health NHS Trust has been offering recovery courses at their recovery college since September 2010. Its aim is for mental health sufferers to become experts in their own care and the courses are run by peer support workers – people with lived experience – and also mental health professionals. The Trust offers courses in 'Planning your own Recovery', 'Leading a Healthy Lifestyle', 'Telling your own Story' and 'Returning to work or Education', as well as a course in 'Taking Back Control'. The latter looks at the situations mental health sufferers find themselves in, how they feel and how they can spot early warning signs in order to avoid relapse and crises. The college has library and computer facilities and encourages students to put in as much as they can.

Indeed, in one study two thirds of students who attended courses here felt they are more able to do the things they want in life, whilst the same amount felt they were able to set the goals they want to achieve in life. Moreover, 80% of students agreed that they now have a plan for how they can stay well or become well.

I have greatly benefited from meeting virtually Mr Jeremy Coutinho, Manager of the Recovery College and Welfare Benefits Team at South West London and St George's Mental Health NHS Trust. He explained that the courses there give an opportunity not only to access additional support and meet others, but they really help the individual to see how different situations and circumstances affect them and how they can detect early warning signs and act accordingly. For me, this may be in taking too much on and getting stressed. It is a different environment from just being seen by a key worker, yet it is a great support to the individual. Ultimately, it is a huge support also to the key workers who manage substantial and difficult case-loads. As I have discussed regarding the 'No Force First' initiative, the main success was about increasing safety. Here, at such a venue as a recovery college, recognising when patients may be feeling unwell or may be starting to feel unwell is a huge step towards reducing relapses and the demand for crisis and in-patient services that are stretched nationwide. It is a win-win situation for all concerned and, with the success that South West London and St George's Mental Health Trust has experienced, it is one which each Trust in the country should seriously consider implementing.

There are also other ways to help those in mental health need. Lincolnshire Partnership NHS Foundation Trust offers accessible online videos for dealing with mental health problems such as stress and anxiety. Their courses focus on different but equally as important angles of mental health; for example, '*Dreaming of a better night's sleep*', '*Letting go of worries*', '*Living more in the moment*' and '*Digital Well-being*' to name just a few. These courses are available to anyone aged 16 years or older in Lincolnshire. Having such a broad range of general mental health courses can also help those who do not have a key worker but may be suffering with milder mental health issues.

Leeds and York Partnership NHS Foundation Trust is currently operating an online recovery course, again similar to South West London and St George's NHS Trust in themes but they also issue newsletters, which include providing information on mental health and social distancing and the implementation of a hub for coronavirus and mental health.

Cambridgeshire and Peterborough NHS Foundation Trust offers a comprehensive list of recovery topics ranging from '*Boundaries*' and '*Risk-taking*' to '*Comfort zones*', '*Recovery Pathway*' and '*Spirituality*'. They operate 'Recovery Coach Teams' which are made up of a recovery coach and peer support workers. These teams cover the Trust's geographical area and they can help towards reducing the need for hospital readmission. However, they have also been favourable to those being discharged from secondary mental healthcare.

One of the main principles is around setting goals and trust and living a satisfying and fulfilling life.

There is much scope to assist not only those in secondary care but also those who may visit their GP. As a wider benefit, co-production could be useful and helpful in GP practices. As a drop-in resource, should there be a need, patients could receive some educational support from a peer support worker. Visiting the GP is often the first port of call when there are early warning signs and having a peer support worker on hand to talk through any triggers could be very beneficial following a GP consultation, should this be agreed in any WRAP (Wellness Recovery Action Plan) plan, as it could enable solutions and a plan to be put in place should these situations reoccur.

Facts And Figures About Recovery Colleges

ImROC has produced a report on recovery colleges. ImROC stands for 'Implementing Recovery through Organisational Change' and they are the organisation which **"Strives for systems, services and cultures to support recovery and wellbeing: locally, nationally and internationally."** They are a not-for-profit organisation which is hosted by Nottinghamshire Healthcare NHS Foundation Trust. There are 85 recovery colleges in the UK with 77 of these being in England; the first recovery college being opened in 2010.

One of the methodologies around recovery is the idea of co-production. This means that the idea of the model is that it is (as previously mentioned) a bottom-up approach and is led primarily by those with lived experiences of mental health illness who are known as peer support workers.

This is essential as for many with mental health concerns, they feel hopeless and the support from their key worker may be somewhat limited. Having someone with lived experiences involved in working in recovery teams and colleges can give tremendous support to someone who is struggling. In this way patients can take on board the experiences of peer support workers who have also suffered detrimental circumstances and can show them how they recovered from them, step by step.

ImROC's study into the success of recovery colleges found that 93% of participants agreed that co-production formed a strong basis in their recovery college.

In terms of recovery colleges having an educational approach, ImROC continues by reporting that 97% of students agreed that education was a fundamental part of their care. Being an educational environment, patients or service users are known as students. They have access to a personal tutor and academic material, provided in an informative and supportive manner. It is crucial that this educational support takes individuals away from the mental health care arena. It offers a structured angle to help those who may otherwise make progress.

Furthermore, Rinaldi and Wybourn (2011) reported that almost 70% of students surveyed 18 months after first attending the college had become mainstream students, gained employment or started volunteering. Rennison et al (2014) and Hall et al (2016), using the social inclusion web, found students reported significant increases in contact with education, employment and volunteering, the arts and social interactions with family and neighbourhoods. Meddings et al (2015) found there were increases in social networks and the number of people students felt able to talk to about mental health and recovery.

The Role of In-House Mental Health Helplines and the Recovery Model

For years, charity helplines geared at supporting the mentally vulnerable have succeeded in bridging gaps in healthcare by providing out-of-hours telephone support. Their function, in helping those in distress or with depressive or other social stressors, has, however, changed in terms of its own internal dynamics. Being listening organisations, their ethos mainly focused on hearing concerns, worries and issues. From my own personal viewpoint, I felt their approach fostered good working relationships and the ability for individuals like myself to feel empowered to take action, no matter what shape or form.

Charity helplines such as the focus line previously run by Rethink have been replaced by in-house NHS mental health helplines. Owing to coronavirus, we have as a nation been fortunate to have 24-hour mental health telephone services. We really could not ask for more. But how does their function relate to the empowerment of patients? Their function is ever improving in its approach to service users in how they empower service users. Being empowered sometimes means the support from someone who shows true belief, yet having the flexibility to support them in the best way possible. Being approachable and non-judgemental, this enables the patient to show true examination and reflection of the situation they find themselves in. Having greater alignment with community teams that are open during core hours of 9am to 5pm, there is peace of mind that support between separate teams is well connected. The service has developed to be one which listens and empathises, crucial for many in times of crisis. This goes hand in hand with a peer to peer service which has proven to empower patients to be (as previously stated) 'peers', moving forwards with their own plans and projects to strive towards their own goals, motivated also by a non-judgemental voice supporting them to take action and progress on their journey.

In-house Trust helplines are highly qualified and helpful – and there appears to be growing scope from my experience to assist the individual in a capacity which empowers them more but which can be more of an albeit 'clinical' aid. Furthermore, as said above, it is my view that helplines that are autonomous from, or now aligned to NHS Trusts are reaching out more to those who may wish a more person-centred approach as opposed to the 'clinician providing health advice to the mental health patient' approach.

So, moving forwards, how can in-house mental health helplines be even more aligned to promote empowerment, self-action and independence? Offering a service which can be fully transparent in its outlook can only assist patients to push themselves forwards in their recovery. Having a holistic, empathetic and non-judgmental approach to patients' needs by listening can, in a mental health helpline setting, demonstrate to patients that they can act and overcome their particular problems. Services that instruct patients, and therefore present restrictions, can deter some from calling and lead to an escalation of issues and further care needs, so it is crucial that there is an apparent system supporting the belief in patients.

The Wider Impact of The Recovery Model On Staffing Within the NHS Mental Health Services

Following a conversation I had with Dave Riley at NHS Merseycare in relation to 'No Force First', I asked Dave about the large amount of money that had been saved by implementing 'No Force First' into the secure in-patient units there in the Liverpool region. I asked specifically whether it had enabled a greater number of personnel to be employed. He replied that while significant funds had been saved, this was not reflected in staff feeling that wards were better staffed but that the wards were and are much safer. It is my view that this demonstrates positively how more staff feel able to spend more time in work and less time off work which, in essence, is what all parties want. Who actually wants to spend most of their employment off sick? If staff feel anxious being at work, this will affect their mental health to such a degree that soon they are unable to attend work.

Having made such tremendous savings from this hugely successful project, there are, of course, most certainly funds available to put further things in place for the staff; for example, chill-out rooms – maybe after a long day at work they could have a few minutes to unwind or a challenging situation may occur which means they need to de-stress.

Recovery colleges in themselves provide a great resource for staff. Not only do they provide community nurses and occupational therapists with a place to refer patients for educational support, they have, as stated, been proven to drastically reduce the number of re-referrals to in-patient services. They enable patients to progress and develop in an educational setting that harnesses their emotional development. Patients need structure. A nurse can't offer 100% of this; some of it needs to come from an educational class. I have attended a peer support recovery group at Nottinghamshire Healthcare Recovery College. There were around 10 students in attendance and the class was led by a Peer Support Advocate. The class covered a topic about the importance of taking responsibility and set down a structure which was very clear and cohesive. These classes are hugely powerful and can propel patients or 'students' on to achieve goals and success in ways that they would otherwise have found quite difficult. So, how does this impact on the case-loads of staff? Some may argue that patients just get fed through the system quicker. As more leave, more come in. Staff are always, therefore, overworked and stressed. If, however, these recovery classes enable many to avoid re-admission, the classes are, therefore, breaking the cycle and are a key component in helping the patient on to a better place in their life. It would be likely, therefore, that reductions in services would happen as a result of implementing educational classes and that should enable at least some freeing up of case-load work and a reduction in risks, at least for some patients previously reliant on the workforce.

It could also be argued that issues surrounding support for staff such as back-fill could be better funded. So, what is back-fill and why has it proven to be such a tall order? It is basically the work cover required for any NHS professional who is on training of any sort. In order for NHS staff to progress, there are a range of options available to them; for example, moving from Support Work to Occupational Therapy. Consequently, back-fill is required for the time this professional is on training, so their duties are covered by a replacement. Not only would the savings from having recovery classes installed within community mental health settings enable scope for patients to receive such education but in having classes for patients, the classes would naturally 'free up' time for nurses and support workers otherwise having busy schedules to attend classes around their chosen training or enable "down time" to get tasks done that otherwise would take longer to do. There would be no need to pay for additional staff at a high price, nor would there be any financial dilemmas for managers who, at the very best of times, often struggle to meet competing demands. Back-fill has often been a contentious issue, so why do we need to look further when the answers are clear?

When our NHS staff are not supported, this can create internal conflict and tremendous job dissatisfaction. If we do not feel able to support those who work tirelessly to help those in their care when we don't see the value that the recovery model brings, it is time to start asking ourselves why we are then complaining about services and budgets being stretched? In developing your organisation, you need to help those in clinical services to be able to better help themselves so this has a knock-on effect on staff so they can further their careers, demonstrating the bottom-up approach of helping patients to explore educational avenues. This means that management staff, too, can feel better equipped and happier to allow staff to receive training and develop further or be able to take time between appointments. Which manager can truly say that they like making difficult decisions that can adversely affect their staff in terms of their morale? Managers would certainly have an easier job when they are aware that staff wishing to be trained can do so more freely and easily. This positive knock-on effect of the recovery model strategies would filter through all layers of each Trust.

The impact of the recovery model on NHS Mental Health Occupational Health Services

Having worked for the NHS mental health service, I was lucky enough to have been supported by the Occupational Health Service. It is a crucial service in helping staff with health problems to return to work on a basis that suits their health needs. Being in heavy demand due to the stressors and pressures that all staff are under, it is no surprise that there are often long waiting times for occupational health services.

NHS staff themselves suffer from a variety of disabilities, often exacerbated by the incredibly intense jobs they do. They are repeatedly pushed to the limit with demand for services and are frequently unable to meet those demands due to deficiencies in staffing. Staff in the health service have their own recovery to deal with, constantly evaluating, learning from situations and assessing how the services they provide can be improved. But can they be improved if there are no free resources or time to enable them to do so?

If, however, the upward pressure exerted on staff, due to unsafe case-loads, high risk situations and increasing demands from a variety of sources, could be reduced by allowing time for training, non-contact time or more special leave as a direct result of enabling recovery classes for patients to take place, this could help ease the pressure that staff face daily. The problems occur because services are so overstretched that those who take time off sick must wait a long time to be seen by Occupational Health. Indeed, Occupational Health staff have high case-loads.

Having regular opportunities to de-stress following stressful occurrences would be beneficial for all. In my previous book, *Mental Health Recovery: Protecting Our Front Line NHS Staff*, I suggested as a solution a chill-out room for staff that they can access quickly and easily following distress. Measures such as this, as well as non-contact time, would not only reduce the demand on Occupational Health Services but would allow staff to take some time for themselves. This is providing, of course, that such relaxation has been enabled as a result of implementing recovery classes.

More Facts and Figures and Information On Recovery Model Savings

I just wanted to pick up on previous figures, notably the financial savings made by Camden and Islington NHS Foundation Trust. As a basis for future financial projections if every NHS mental health trust bought 15 self-contained flats for patients who were at risk of readmission the savings could be enormous. Given that there are 54 NHS mental health trusts in the United Kingdom, each one could potentially be looking at similar savings of £440,000. This equates to a total possible saving of £23,760,000 across the UK. In Year 2 of operation, this could save this vital part of the NHS in excess of £47,520,000. Moreover, following NHS Merseycare's example could see the same number of NHS mental health trusts save a funding total in excess of £13,446,000 in sickness absence costs in Year 1 across all 54 trusts, more or less doubling to £26,892,000 in Year 2. While there would also be costs in training staff on 'No Force First', these would be largely set-up costs that would decrease as more staff are trained and, hopefully, retained on the in-patient wards.

Bearing in mind that these are just two strategies, there are many more savings that the recovery model itself possesses. An economic analysis of the work done at South West London and St George's Mental Health NHS Trust's recovery college has yet to be completed, although the strong evidence that Jeremy Coutinho passed on to me shows that as the majority of patients had moved on, following the recovery classes offered to education, voluntary work and paid work, this evidence suggests the bottom-up approach not only helps patients to progress with their lives but also reduces some of the burden on secondary mental health and in-patient services. This shows clearly, therefore, that at least some of those who had received in-patient and secondary care were either not requiring the same level of support or requiring it to a lesser degree having attended a set of classes there. This, in turn, could suggest that clinicians could see a reduction in case-loads and hospital readmission, allowing them to help those in more acute need.

How Can the Recovery Model Be Applied to Other NHS Mental Health Services? – Eating Disorders

Many NHS Trusts also look after adults and children with eating disorders. As per the MIND web page, an eating disorder is ***"portrayed as a desire to be the thinnest person in the world for vanity purposes."*** There are strict criteria for many eating disorder services and there are often waiting lists. Making the patient the expert by empowering them to help others on a peer-to-peer basis could be hugely beneficial so any patient is aware that someone has been in their shoes and has successfully come out of the other side. It is a belief challenge that could be bolstered by having fellow peer workers to support those on a one-to-one basis. This would impact positively on the patient concerned as they would know that someone really understands inside out what they are going through.

Indeed, Beat, the leading charity for eating disorders in the UK, reports that: *"Families currently do not receive adequate support in looking after a loved one with an illness that can consume their own energy and family life as well as the health of the sufferer. Sofia, a mother, described a situation faced by many parents: "We get no respite, whatsoever…I've been on pretty much 24/7 duty, looking after her for the last four or five years, really. We have had no respite from that, whatsoever, and there's nothing [to help us." Another mother, Victoria, admitted that 'both of us were really falling apart."*

Beat also states the following: *"Beat seeks to address this by calling on all healthcare providers to adopt eight best practice standards, encouraging them to:*

1. *Have a policy that ensures optimum involvement of and support for all carers as soon as a loved one starts treatment.*
2. *Train all service staff in the application of the policy and these standards with particular focus on the importance of carers as a resource for recovery.*
3. *Provide all carers with useful and comprehensive information about eating disorders when their loved one receives a diagnosis.*
4. *Offer all carers and siblings an assessment of their own needs when a loved one receives an eating disorder diagnosis, continue to monitor their wellbeing throughout the sufferer's treatment and, where necessary, refer carers to specialist services.*
5. *Offer all carers options for peer-to-peer support.*
6. *Offer all carers opportunities to learn the necessary skills to provide optimum support for their loved ones.*
7. *Inform and engage carers when a loved one faces a transition between services and ensure that effective communication between both services and carers takes place.*
8. *Provide a mechanism by which carers' input and feedback is sought and acted upon."*

Furthermore, there is evidence which suggests that, in using peer support workers, following the principles of the recovery model does help to improve the lives of those suffering with eating disorders.

The US National Library of Medicine and National Institute of Health published the following extract from the Journal of Eating Disorders:

"The peer support intervention was designed to run concurrently with the hospital program with focus on removing the additional barriers to recovery, such as low motivation for recovery that are not specifically targeted by traditional health systems. Participant groups of inpatients, day-patients and outpatients each attended two structured group sessions and completed pre- and post-group questionnaires. Quantitative and qualitative analyses comparing pre to post-group ratings revealed a significant decrease in participant's feelings of stigma associated with having an eating disorder; a significant increase in hope and motivation for recovery and a better future and improved trust and acceptance of the hospital treatment they were currently receiving."

Having an Eating Disorder Peer Support Worker, albeit on a voluntary basis could not only give purpose to those who have suffered but also help clinicians treating those who are unwell by supporting their work. Again, here it could be expected that cases would, as a result, be less prolonged and eating disorder champion work, as part of the recovery model, could be done in schools, universities and self-help support groups linked to or independent of the NHS. It would, of course, act as a big confidence boost to the peer support worker or champion.

So, in the wider context with more recovery and preventative work there could be a vast reduction in cases and shortened treatment plans. With education comes knowledge and therefore savings. Those who can learn from others are more likely to achieve a full recovery and those educated in advance may not require further assistance.

This is good news for the NHS but it's also extremely good news for those in need or in potential need. Prevention, as we know, is better than cure but the recovery model shows us that someone needing help can get 'out of the hole' much quicker and easier with a peer support worker as opposed to a patient being treated solely by a clinician. Shouldn't we explore other avenues that could greatly help those who are in need or at potential risk in order to avoid unhappiness? Isn't providing additional cost-effective resources justifiable to help those who are suffering to recover more quickly, as well as lowering spikes in demand for services?

Drugs And Alcohol Services

Peer support in drugs and alcohol services is already very prevalent. Many support workers who were previously addicts act as amazing peer workers, given their experience and their ability to fully empathise with those suffering the addictions. As well as NHS services, there are institutions who actively promote the importance of peer support in helping these ones recover from such addictions. Having someone who has had similar experiences and been able to overcome them can really provide assurance to those who may have developed mental health conditions as a result of illicit substance abuse that these addictions can be beaten.

There is also often a link between mental ill health and drug and alcohol addiction. Many develop mental health concerns as a result of taking drugs and excessive alcohol. Many, too, develop mental ill health, such as depression and use drugs or alcohol to compensate for this low mood and anxiety. Situations can arise that push people to take illicit substances in order to cope, while there are times when mental ill health itself can cause many to turn to such negative coping mechanisms.

The Priory Hospital in North London believes that peer support, as part of their addiction programme, is essential to the recovery of those admitted to its care as it offers strength, hope and encouragement to these ones.

Indeed, one such review on their website is detailed below which clearly corroborates this:

"Is this what recovery looks like?"

"Can't be right. This bloke seems pretty well-adjusted. Relaxed. Clear, smiling eyes. Is this what recovery looks like?"

That's what I thought about the first peer supporter I remember seeing. There would have been others before him. But I was orbiting Pluto for a few days and too absorbed in myself to notice or care.

Then I started to pay attention. And it was this chap, who voluntarily gave up his time, that set me on my way to thinking 'maybe I could change too'. Why not?

I enjoyed the daily 12-Step meetings and the sense of connection and belonging they gave me. And, of course, the

'chairs' of the meeting were illuminating – be it their pain, tragedy, humour or hope. However, the peer supporters that I 'gelled with', gave me something extra: a deeper, more personal insight into how recovery had changed their lives.

Who were these people and why did they choose to walk into the lion's den and face a room full of patients who'd spent the day pouring out their darkest moments (or not) and facing some harsh realities and who now probably just wanted to chill out and watch X Factor?

Tough gig for anyone – but they just rolled with it. The answer was surprisingly easy: they'd been there, done it, come out the other side, and wanted to give back.

I decided then, that I wanted to do peer support. I thought of it as a benchmark for the success of my recovery. On reflection, I think that was my ego talking. Maybe. Maybe not. I don't really care. I do peer support now and believe that it comes from a good place.

I'm fortunate enough to support a therapist every week in an aftercare session with ex-patients and do a monthly one-hour talk that includes a Q&A. It's the Q&A that I enjoy the most. You don't get the opportunity to do that in a 12-Step meeting but here you can really get to grips with what's going on with the patients and let the session flow.

My approach to the talks is to be 'normal'. I just say it how it was for me and how it is now. I don't preach. I don't assume the guys have intimate knowledge of the 12 steps, nor do I ram them home – I contextualise them and give evidence on how they worked for me. I discuss how a step, or something I learned on the Addiction Treatment Programme, connects to my work life, social life, inner life, family life and so on.

I've done quite a few talks in the last six years and I've learned that it's important to make patients feel comfortable. The more relaxed they are, the more they listen and the more they ask. I don't blast in there with jokes but I do use humour liberally – if it feels right. I guess that's it; with experience, one gets to quickly assess the mood of the room and the approach to take.

It's also vital to keep the room moving. Over time, I've learned techniques to gently close down dominant voices and ensure everyone can have their say – should they choose to. Occasionally, difficult subjects come up where I have asked the patient to raise it with a therapist. When handled carefully, I've found the group is generally supportive in these instances.

I also feel a special bond with other peer supporters. We meet regularly and have the opportunity to share anything that's on our minds (we are encouraged to process anything that may be triggering with a therapist or a peer). There's honesty and great camaraderie in these sessions – I think it's more than us having a shared experience and, if you will, surviving. I think the common denominator is compassion. Hard-won compassion.

I talk a lot about responsibility. It's not a classic recovery or therapeutic concept, but it's one of the biggest messages I have to pass on. Responsibility is at the core of my life now. I take responsibility for my actions and I behave in a responsible way. That doesn't mean I don't have fun – far from it!

I've learned that the more responsible I am; the more freedom I have. And the more freedom I have, the more I want to use it responsibly. Realistically, my mind can't

handle unlimited freedom. It couldn't while fizzing on drugs or flying on booze and it can't clean and sober. It was a myth. Responsibility gives me a workable boundary in which to fully engage with life and, depending on what's been thrown at me, I can cope or thrive.

Part of this responsibility is a healthy commitment to peer support. Not out of duty or loyalty to Priory or the patients. I do it because it feels like the right thing to do and I enjoy the warm feeling when connecting with someone for the first time or seeing a glimmer of hope rising.

I recently re-read the promises I'd made to myself on my first day at Priory. Under the section 'what do I want to achieve?' I'd scrawled just one sentence in capitals: "To get the twinkle back in my eye. Well, the twinkle is well and truly back and long may it remain."

This extract confirms that the role of peer support in the rehabilitation of drug and alcohol addictions is pivotal in achieving a high success rate for those seeking help. Being able to reason with those who require help and support and to explain the benefits of acting responsibly in a constructive environment is a strategy that is extremely beneficial. Learning from one another is crucial and learning from someone who has been in a similar situation takes away blame, guilt and judgement.

While it may be difficult to see how peer support can play a role in child and adolescent mental health, given that some strategies will not help children, it is clear that recovery strategies are vital in helping the young to express their feelings and circumvent difficulties that arise. For example, showing how adult role models overcome depression can really have a powerful impact on a child's recovery.

Derbyshire Healthcare NHS Foundation Trust demonstrate how peer support as an integral part of the recovery model can provide empathy for children. On their web page they present clear examples to children by the use of celebrities, which enables them to relate to what is being communicated:

"We are all different and no one's journey in life is the same. But sometimes reading about other people's experiences can help us. It shows that we are not alone and that things can and do get better."

Anyone can experience mental health difficulties and this includes celebrities! Check out some of their stories below…

Davina McCall

Davina says: "Talking about mental health problems should be as easy as talking about physical health problems – you wouldn't be ashamed or scared to tell someone you were ill would you? Being open about mental health goes a long way to breaking down the stigma. It's time to talk, it's Time to Change."

J.K. Rowling

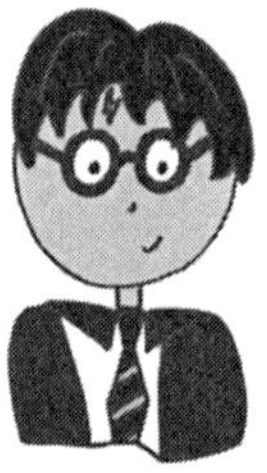

One of the most famous writers in the world shows that mental health problems do not have to stop you from doing things in your life. J.K. Rowling used writing to help with her depression and through this found world fame!

John Green

Famous for writing 'The Fault in Our Stars', John Green has spoken openly in the media about his struggles with anxiety and OCD (obsessive compulsive disorder) and the treatment he has received for this. Showing his fans that they are not alone.

…And there's more

See a list of celebrity mental health supporters at: www.time-to-change.org.uk/news-media/celebrity-supporters

Leanne's story

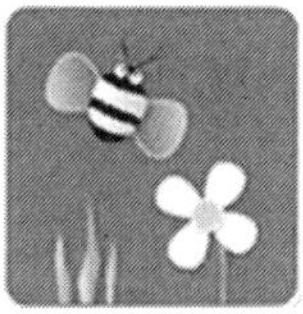

Leanne is a young person from Derbyshire who has been supported by our CAMHS team. Here, she explains why it's so important to talk about mental health.

Mental Health is nothing to be ashamed of. Just like physical health, it is something we all have and sometimes in our life we struggle with it, some more than others.

It was hard as a young person with poor mental health, especially at school; I felt very misunderstood. My peers struggled to understand my behaviour and why for example I found speaking in front of the class a hard thing to do. Until more recent years, anxiety had such a tight grip on my life, I found going out to meet friends hard, getting buses near-on impossible and making decisions was a task I dreaded. Anxiety impacted my life so much that I wasn't the person I dreamed to be. Inside, I was a whole different me.

People said all kinds of unhelpful things like 'you need to get over this.' Sometimes I felt they thought I wanted to be the way I was. I couldn't see things being any other way or changing. I felt so trapped in a world I didn't want to be in, that I didn't go as far as planning for tomorrow, I didn't

see much point. My family and friends struggled to understand me and I struggled to help myself.

I now see that I so badly needed care, support, time and love and I did receive these things in the form of an amazing teacher, counselling, therapy and brilliant friendships. It was the people who gave me these things that really helped me to turn my life around. They didn't just help me change my life, they saved me from myself.

I now am open about my experiences in the hope that for other people this will give them the small nudge to be open about their own, to realise that sometimes, it's okay not to be ok and to seek help if this is necessary. Seeking help is everything but weakness, it takes courage to stand and look at yourself.

Suffering from a mental illness at a young age is frightening and especially so without knowing that others have suffered too, how to seek help or what to do to make it better. It can affect the way children communicate, affect their appetite and make them resist social distractions, yet with the right support from a recovery model base can really assist recovery among children.

Family Health

Families play a central role in supporting those who experience mental health difficulties. Indeed, my family have been a pinnacle of support: when they came frequently to see me in hospital in the year 2000 to all the support at home and while I was at university where there was much stress and strain. Not only have I been lucky enough to receive emotional and financial support, I have also, as a result, been motivated to keep well and on the correct path. Families are often multiple sources of support, including practical, financial and emotional. Who can say that they have never turned to a family member for help of some sort? It is, however, not just offspring who suffer with mental health issues. Parents also are often faced with multiple stressors, for example, paying mortgages, rent and bills as well as other worries, and the concern for their children's welfare and this can result in them suffering depression or more severe mental health difficulties. Family Focused Practice (FFP) (Maybery, D and Reupert, A) has also recently been applied to families where one or both parents suffer mental health concerns:

"FFP is a collaborative approach that encompasses both the individual and his or her family (Rosenbaum et al, 1998). The principles of FFP were foremost developed from a review of the literature by Allen and Petre (1998) and have been expanded since (Dempsey and Keen, 2008; Dunst et al, 2007). These principles are summarised as follows:

1. ***Family is central to the lives of individuals. This means identifying the family as a unit of intervention rather than the individual with the presenting 'problem'.***
2. ***Maximising families' choices and abilities for informed decision-making rather than a professional centric model of decision-making. This acknowledges that parents know their children best,***

know what is best for their children and have ultimate care for their children.

3. ***Applying a strengths-based perspective, as opposed to a deficit or pathological perspective of the family. Rather than 'blame' the family, practitioners need to recognise that all families have strengths that can be further developed and used in problem solving.***
4. ***Recognising that all families are different and will require culturally competent services that value diversity and multiple perspectives."***

Maybery and Reupert continue to explain how the family unit supports each member's mental health:

"While often described as an individual journey, recovery is increasingly recognised as a relational concept, where the social environment, in particular one's family, is critical (Reupert et al, 2015a, b). A crucial aspect of any recovery model is support for an individual's choices including his or her choice about being a parent."

Nicholson (2014) also adds that the recovery model can show support and strength for parents, as well as children:

There are several links between parenting and recovery that have only recently been documented. For example, Nicholson (2014) found that children may give parents the strength and will to 'keep going' thereby promoting hope, a key recovery component. 'Being a parent' and effectively assuming the parenting role provide parents with meaning and purpose, another element of recovery (Maybery et al,

2015). Parenting may also give opportunities for meaningful interactions and activities and connections into their community (Maybery et al, 2015). Thus, identifying and supporting an individual's parenting role can provide hope, a sense of agency, connectedness, self-determination and meaning, all cognisant with a recovery approach.

Perinatal Services

Perinatal services, too, highlight another area where recovery work is prominent, and the concerns of those women who suffer during pregnancies are explained below by NHS England:

"Perinatal mental health (PMH) problems are those which occur during pregnancy or in the first year following the birth of a child. Perinatal mental illness affects up to 20% of new and expectant mums and covers a wide range of conditions.

If left untreated, mental health issues can have significant and long-lasting effects on the woman, the child and the wider family. Specialist PMH services provide care and treatment for women with complex mental health needs and support the developing relationship between parent and baby. They also offer women with mental health needs advice for planning a pregnancy."

Perinatal services are closely linked with other mental health services, such as secondary care and IAPT services, for example. Patients are referred into their service from other key mental health services, yet, in terms of the help which is offered, these services and others may serve as a point of being referred back to or accessed simultaneously. The work that they do reflects the principles of the recovery model, in ***"Educating and supporting the individual (and meaningful others) to be aware of triggers for illness and the development of resilience and coping strategies."*** (Miller, Clinical: The recovery approach to life-changing conditions)

Indeed, the benefits of the work that perinatal departments offer encompassing the recovery model can be summarised as the following:

"-Improving recovery rates and outcomes for women and their children, including reducing the risk of adverse psychological, social, parenting and employment outcomes

-Reducing the risk of premature births and stillbirths, obstetric complications and delayed physical growth in the developing baby

-Reducing the risk of behavioural and emotional problems for the child later in life and the likelihood of lower IQ and lower educational attainment

-Reducing wider societal costs – of the £8.1 billion described above, almost £6 billion relates to the impact on the child rather than the mother."

Wider Benefits of The Recovery Model in the Community – Crime

Teaching patients about how to look after themselves and others is an important tool that can help some to avoid taking the wrong path. Many who have been imprisoned because of crimes committed often also have mental health worries. Many repeatedly turn to crime to fund the expense of taking drugs, which then results in negative consequences and, in turn, does not help their mental health. Many also commit offences to fund drugs having previously been diagnosed with a mental health condition in order for them to blank out any difficult emotional circumstances.

The positive implications of the recovery model on crime are also huge. Educational settings that support those at an early stage can provide a structure and help steer some away from following paths they had previously taken. Many who feel that society has rejected them or who have had traumatic childhoods or relationship breakdowns can all benefit from a positive influence. Many have never had the kind of education or support that some Healthcare Trusts offer. Giving people a sense of purpose, positive goals can be created and hope of recovery restored. Educational classes, whilst having some educational cost, have so many vast benefits. Having been proven to have a positive impact for mental health purposes and avenues of hope, it would be perfectly plausible to suggest that they could also have a positive impact on helping to reduce crime.

Police forces across the country deal with the mentally ill on a regular basis. Many forces feel they often do not have the appropriate resources to look after those who require specialist help. Left with no alternative, they may have to leave many vulnerable patients locked up in police cells until they can be properly assessed. The Police must often help in such situations that may re-occur and they may themselves lack the training in how to deal with the mentally disadvantaged. The following is an extract from Zoë Billingham at Her Majesty's Inspectorate of Constabulary and Fire and Rescue Service:

"The last resort, not the first port of call.

In our inspection, we found that the police approach to people with mental health problems is generally supportive, considerate and compassionate. But we believe there is only so much the police can do to improve the overall picture. This is because, in our view, too many aspects of the broader mental health system are broken; the police are left to pick up the pieces. The fact that almost every police force now has its own mental health triage team indicates that there isn't nearly enough emphasis on early intervention and primary care to prevent the need for a crisis response. This is letting down people with mental health problems, as well as placing an intolerable burden on police officers and staff. It is a national crisis which should not be allowed to continue; there needs to be a fundamental rethink and urgent action. People with mental health problems need expert support. Those in crisis need to be cared for in a healthcare setting. They shouldn't be locked in a police cell or held for hours on end in the back of a police car for their own safety. This expert help needs to be available whenever people need it; mental health crises don't just happen during office hours. All too often, the system is failing people when they most need help. This is not a problem that the police alone can solve. Other services need to stop relying on the 24/7 availability of the police. We have grave concerns about whether the police should be involved in responding to mental health problems to the degree they are. Our

inspection found that,] in dealing with people with mental health problems, police officers and staff must do complex and high-risk work. They often don't have the skills they need to support people with mental health problems. And, too often, they find themselves responsible for the safety and welfare of people that other professionals would be better placed to deal with. This means that already overstretched and all-too-often overwhelmed police officers can't always respond appropriately and people in mental health crisis don't always get the help they need. All this can take a heavy emotional toll on officers and staff. This isn't about blaming either the police or mental health practitioners. We recognise the considerable work that all services and agencies have done to improve the response to those with mental health problems. But in our view, the emphasis overall needs to be far more on early intervention and community care. As HM Chief Inspector of Constabulary, Sir Thomas Winsor, said in his 2017 State of Policing report: "There will always be situations where someone in crisis needs a rapid response from the emergency services. But too often, our public services are failing to work together to prevent the crisis in the first place…blue lights should not have to flash for someone to get the help they need in time." There are a few things the police could do better. They could give officers and staff better mental health training and have a clearer view of the level of demand from people with mental health problems. We have made some recommendations along these lines which could help improve their approach. However, these can only go so far and there needs to be a longer-term solution. When it

comes to mental ill-health, the police should be the last resort, not the first port of call."

Zoë Billingham, HM Inspector of Constabulary

From the extract, it is clear to me that more work needs to be done to try to prevent the escalation of mental ill health. How do we let it get to such urgent stages? Early intervention work, as described by Ms Billingham, could help many to avoid recurrent episodes where the Police also need to step in and help to resolve difficulties. The recovery model provides answers to the concerns the Police have by providing training where necessary but also enabling many who have been through system to experience an alternative approach and learn new things about themselves. Indeed, there is evidence from the Ministry of Justice's report into "Transforming Rehabilitation – a summary of evidence on reducing offending" which shows what factors contribute to reoffending and what solutions there are. Although the report is ambiguous, there are lessons to be learnt on how recovery strategies could help to steer many away from reoffending:

"Although offenders are not a homogeneous group, a range of problems or needs are more frequently observed in offender populations than in the general population. These include substance misuse problems, pro-criminal attitudes, difficult family backgrounds including experience of childhood abuse or time spent in care, unemployment and financial problems, homelessness and mental health problems. Many of these factors are interlinked. They will vary from individual to individual and group to group, for instance by gender and age."

Again, the report provides answers by breaking down what factors help criminals to stop reoffending, or to "desist":

Desistance Factor	Link to Desistance
Getting older and maturing	Getting older and maturing tend to support desistance, particularly for those involved in street crime where, typically, offending rates peak in the late teens or early 20s, then decline steadily before dropping off sharply around the age of 30. This may be due to ex-offenders giving more attention to their families and relationships (see below). The likelihood of reoffending after release from custody reduces with age.
Family and relationships	There is evidence that forming strong and supportive intimate bonds with others appears to help desistance from crime, although more contemporary research is needed on this subject. Family and such relationships can reduce the amount of time spent in groups of same-age, same-sex friends (a known risk factor for young male offending). Strong partnerships and relationships with his or her children also provide an individual with something to lose if there is a return to prison. Living with non-offending parents can have the same sort of effect on ex-offenders who have returned to the family home. Finally, family and

	intimate attachments may give offenders a sense of purpose, meaning and direction. Individuals who devote themselves to raising their children or caring for elderly parents may find that crime and imprisonment are incompatible with such roles.
Sobriety	Drug and alcohol dependency and misuse are associated with offending. Recovery from addiction is often a key part of desistance processes, although the effect is not automatic, and some individuals may abstain from addictive substances but not crime or vice versa.
Employment	Evidence suggests that steady employment – particularly if it offers a sense of achievement, satisfaction or mastery – can support offenders in stopping offending. Employment has been identified as an important factor in supporting desistance among offenders aged over 27. However, employment alone cannot prevent offending and some offenders can desist without employment.
Hope and motivation	Research suggests that individuals who desist from crime are usually very motivated and confident that they can change their lives: offenders who clearly say they want to stop offending are the most likely to desist. The impact of these motivational factors has even been found in long-term

	studies up to ten years after release from prison.
Having something to give to others	People who feel and show concern and empathy for others are more likely to desist from crime. Offenders who find ways to contribute to society, their community or their families appear to be more successful at giving up crime. If these achievements are formally recognised, the effect may be even stronger.
Having a place within a social group	Those who feel connected to others in a (non-criminal) community are more likely to stay away from crime. Social networks that help desistance include extended family, mutual aid groups, clubs and cultural or religious groups
Not having a criminal identity	People with criminal records who do not define themselves purely as 'offenders' but see themselves as basically good people who made a mistake may find it easier to desist.
Being believed in	Research with those who desist has identified that having someone believe in them is important and that desistance can be supported by interactions with others who communicate a belief that they can and will change, that they are good people and that they have something to offer society or other people."

As previously stated, many of the desistance factors are linked and interwoven which, when broken, can lead to a breakdown and possible negative repercussions. However, more importantly there are many 'bits' of this 'jigsaw puzzle' which are covered by recovery work. For example, having hope and motivation to build a better life makes any individual more likely to desist. Recovery classes cover such topics and are a key focus point to help students realise that they can improve their current situations holistically. If none of us have hope, there is no chance that we can be motivated to make important changes in our lives. Moreover, 'being believed in' is a key component of recovery work. Students who attend recovery classes may lack confidence or may have suffered circumstances that have made them doubt themselves. It may have been from stress at work or a bereavement or, indeed, from crimes committed previously, to name just a few possible scenarios.

Having peers who support one another greatly improves self-worth and shows everyone that they can change and offer society a positive input.

Wider Benefits of The Recovery Model in The Community – General Practice And Other NHS Trusts

Having worked with the local Clinical Commissioning Group to find ways and gaps where things can go wrong for patients, it is apparent that many doctors are often faced with making difficult decisions daily. How can the recovery model help them and the patients they attend to?

Being able to refer patients to an educational course setting would provide general practitioners (GP's) with practical reference support, particularly as they are the first port of call for many who may be new to that area, have no family or friends nearby or may be socially vulnerable. Like courses in Cognitive Behavioural Therapy, courses that are offered, for example at South West London and St George's Mental Health NHS Trust, enable GP's to provide all relevant information as a back-up to their skills and treatments. GP's would benefit from self-training, which I feel would be best placed by GPs attending peer support workshops and sessions.

Not only can GP's learn from these classes, they can also adopt a peer-to-peer recovery initiative that 'practices what they preach', where each GP supports one another, in groups, on a regular basis, on decision-making, treatments and many other related subjects. This is not about telling professionals how to 'suck eggs' but it is to act as a reminder of ways that they can further help one another and relate the recovery model to their own working practices and needs. The NHS GP Health Service Practitioner Health Programme document extract below explains more about this:

Our vision

"All GPs and GP trainees to have access to reflective practice and peer support in groups, which can support their mental wellbeing and contribute to continuous professional development. We believe that by offering GPs and GP trainees an opportunity to meet as a group to have the space and time to reflect and discuss, this will support cultural change in GPs behaviour that becomes an 'everyday' occurrence for 'everyone'. Meeting as a group will support well-being and mental health. GPs who take the time to talk

together, learn from one another, share experiences and support one another in this way will naturally build their resilience and grow their armoury for dealing with the day to day stresses of life in the NHS. The groups can choose any reflective practice modality which allows GPs to meet with their peers for at least 90 minutes in a protected, facilitated space. Each 90 mins as well as enabling some important 'downtime' represents 90 minutes of reflection on your practice, recognised as a key part of your CPD. The Group Peer Support (GPS) scheme will be implemented over the next five years. The concept The NHS Practitioner Health Programme and more recently NHS GP Health Service are aimed at those GPs who become mentally unwell. However, we believe that it is important that all GPs are supported to stay well and have the opportunity to learn and develop the techniques, as a part of CPD, to maintain their own wellbeing and have the time and space to do this. This should form an essential part of their individual continuous professional practice and development. There is evidence that GPS peer support groups, including Balint, reflective practice groups, action learning sets, 'young' practitioner groups and other interventions where doctors (and other staff) come together improves morale, reduces burn out and contributes towards lifelong learning; but currently there is little time in the working day of GPs to come together for periods of reflection, peer support or peer learning. GPS will support GPs to find this time. We wish to work with GPs to develop around 50 GP peer support groups across England (PHP/GPH only have a remit for England) to understand the value and impact that 90 minutes of facilitated peer support can provide. The group attendees

will be asked to complete some basic demographics and contribute to an evaluation process to support the development of the principle on a wide-scale basis."

The Recovery Model and Work

Work has always been a very important factor for me. I graduated in 2005 with a degree in French/Hispanic studies. While university was an incredible achievement for me, the world of work brought with it a whole host of other challenges. Finding a supportive environment and work/life balance is not easy and can present issues for those who do not have underlying health conditions. For those who do have health conditions, like myself, there has been concern over being stable in lasting employment without the need for intermittent breaks. As I was conditioned to work full-time to start with, I found the pressure too overbearing. Yet, I was 'conditioned' to find work in stressful environments. I have worked in a variety of settings and found things tough a lot of the time. I do now claim financial support and my current work as a part-time sales negotiator does suit me better. Why is this the case for me? Well, having a job that is a few days here and a few days there, for me, is very different to a job where you attend every day without a break. The 'breaks' away from work act as a support for me, while the work itself is new and varied, therefore I do not feel as though things become stagnant.

The Scottish Recovery Network 'Pippa Coutts, Scottish Development Centre for Mental Health' (October 2007) issued the following summary about how work can help assist those into recovery:

"Supporting recovery for people with long-term mental health problems includes providing people with choices and opportunities for social development and self-determination. One such opportunity, which mental health service users have requested is for improved support to gain and retain work and employment. Employment is linked to recovery in several ways. For example, the processes that people, who may have been out of work for some time, engage in as they move back to work are often recovery processes, like building self-esteem, self-understanding and motivation. Employment can work to promote recovery through providing people with purpose and structure and through providing opportunities for individuals to give back and contribute to society or individuals. Work is often linked to our identity and therefore healthy employment can have a positive effect on recovery, as can the social networks a job may bring. Not just any work or employment will support recovery, it needs to be the right work for that person, and within a workplace which is flexible and supportive."

Indeed, this is supported by a statement from the Royal College of Psychiatrists who have stated:

"Work is important in promoting the recovery of those who have experienced mental health problems." (RCP, 2003, p5)

I was able to access significant amounts of support in gaining work; in my area I was able to access support from Shaw Trust and Derbyshire Employment Project. Both offered excellent support in job hunting, preparing for interviews, building confidence and follow-ups. It was particularly important for me to have this support as I had left previous jobs on ill-health grounds and felt lost at the best of times. The support was regular and it helped to keep me focused and grounded on making positive steps forward into work. It took me quite some time to get a new job, given the fierce competition, but having consistent support enabled me to feel assured that getting a new job could be achieved. Further to this, the Scottish Recovery Network states:

"The experience of individuals and mental health employability projects around entering work is that when you have or have had a mental health problem the journey back to work can be a long one, where a variety of supports are required at different points on the way. Durie highlights this in the employment matrix, which divides the pathway into a four-part continuum, starting with personal development and moving through support into work, to support in work (2005). The services linked to people's development tend to support recovery through focusing on building confidence, a sense of self-worth and motivation."

In my case, as perhaps with others, work can be a grave source of stress which can, in turn, upset mood and cause distress and, later, subsequent depression. Workplace politics can get in the way of enabling those more vulnerable and mentally more vulnerable to feel comfortable in work, less anxious and more able to contribute effectively:

"Factors beyond the individual, related to wider society and the community, such as friends, family and workplaces act as barriers or facilitators to people's recovery. So supportive and suitable employment can work to recovery through these mechanisms too."

"For employment to effectively promote recovery it needs to be the right kind of employment in the right kind of work place and environment. The workplace factors which promote recovery and promote mental health and wellbeing at work will be considered in the penultimate section."

(RCP, 2003; SRN, 2006; Brown and Kandirikirira, 2007)

Work can be a very positive place to meet new people and socially connect. I have made friends as a result of places I have worked and, while there have been occasions when I have clashed with work colleagues, there have been some very positive encounters also. Work can be a double-edged sword, yet being motivated to try new jobs is crucial if we are to find more meaningful employment:

"Also, employment activity provides opportunities for people to increase their connection to communities around them, which promotes recovery. Employment or other work and social activities can support people to build up their social networks, giving people more chances to meet new people beyond their closest friends and family. The SRN investigation reported that the social nature of work played

a part in many people's recovery." (Brown and Kandirikirira, 2007)

"Promoting access to work for people with mental health problems requires meeting people where they are at and supporting them through their recovery and work aspirations. The evidence from Braitman and colleagues suggests that for people to be successful in finding work, they need to want to work. (Secker et al, 2006) This was the finding of the evaluation of Restart: that the most common individual factor underlying peoples' success in finding work through the project was being ready to enter the process of gaining work." (Bailey et al, 2007)

Throughout the last 15 years I have tried various jobs and had major setbacks along the way. I am by no means 'Superman', and would not like to insinuate that I am in any way better than any other person. I have always tried to look forwards, not backwards, and have hope that I will find my way and move closer towards more suitable work. For me, nothing could be worse than dwelling on experiences that dragged me down when there are possible openings that may work out better. I do think about bad experiences – we all do – but the only thing I can say is that each experience helps us learn and move to something potentially more beneficial:

"Recovery is seen as building hope and a belief in one's self. It has been pointed out that health services and professionals could facilitate service users' employment through presenting more positive messages about their abilities and aspirations regarding work. (Brown and

Kandirikirira, 2007) Currently, people entering mental health services are often told they are unlikely to work again and professionals have tended to either assume service users are not employable or just not put any effort into finding ways of supporting work aspirations. (RCP, 2003) For example, in one study, Rinaldi (2000) found 44% of people with mental health problems who had been successful in accessing employment had been told they would never work again."

I have often found that mental health in the workplace is viewed as a problem, not a strength. Focusing on people's weaknesses does nothing for their self-esteem, nor does it help to unite the workplace, maintaining a supportive environment. From my experiences, there is certainly much work to be done to help support those who may struggle in the workplace. I have been told, "*You won't cope*," or have otherwise not been consulted about adjustments or adjustments which I have requested to be implemented have not been considered. There is a 'back-covering' and box-ticking culture which very often overshadows what would support or would really help the individual. Why is this the case? Often workloads and pressure do not create the space to allow for positive feedback or, perhaps, constructive criticism. But to really help those who are potentially vulnerable in the workplace we need to look closely and carefully at the measures we are implementing: who are they benefiting and for what purpose?

Recovery As a Strengths-Based Approach

The work produced by the Scottish Recovery Network has again produced some examples of how a strengths-based approach can provide the foundations for showing strengths, skills and abilities between worker and patient:

"Like all models and approaches the strengths-based approach has its own assumptions and beliefs. One of these is that: People have strengths, skills and abilities. Strengths based practice uses these skills and personal strengths as the platform on which recovery will be built. Strengths based practitioners do not deny that serious symptoms and problems exist. Suffering, problems, mental distress, and severe difficulties do exist but they are not the whole story."

"The basic principles commence right from the outset. The stance during assessment is yes to empathically explore the problems difficulties and hurdles facing the individual and the greater these problems are, the more amazing it is that the person can be here today to voluntarily participate in assessment at all. This participation alone points to hope and optimism and tells the strengths-based practitioner that the person is willing to engage (as much as they can, given their circumstances) in the process of change. As with all good interventions, the active ingredient is empathy, and so the worker must spend time understanding the person's difficulties and problems and acknowledge vulnerabilities and losses. This process builds rapport and engagement and is experienced by service users as genuinely helpful and supportive.

WORKER AS EXPERT	***WORKER AS CLIENT/COLLABORATOR***
Thinks in terms of problems and mental illness	***Thinks in terms of solutions and mental health***
Use of technical expert language	***Uses persons language and metaphors***
Use of diagnostic labels Pathologies	***Aware of labelling and avoids it De-pathologies.***
Can set goals unilaterally	***Co-constructs goals***
Can impose interventions	***Negotiates joint action plans***
Thinks illness is 'severe and enduring'	***Recognises that recovery is a real possibility***

Nonetheless, from a strengths-based standpoint one of the assessment questions that the worker is very curious about is 'how did you survive all of that to be here today?' In exploring theses survival and coping skills the strengths based approach seeks to unpack and amplify these skills in ever greater detail 'and what else do you do that helps you deal with these problems?' and 'what else?' drawing out the details of the persons problem solving strategies and other resources so that imperceptibly the dialogue between worker and service user takes on the aspect of a curious worker seeking to understand how the expert client manages to deal with whatever mental health or other problems they may have.

Assessment is conducted in a conversational and engaging manner, and the language used to document it, is from the service users' perspective and in their own words, paying attention to the metaphors and images used by the client. Strengths based assessment is viewed as ongoing and evolving. This leads to another key feature of a strengths based, solution-oriented approach, the explicit recognition that the client is the expert. This approach respects and honours the individuals lived experience and involves the worker in relinquishing the role of expert or teacher in favour of that of collaborator working towards recovery in partnership with the service user. This allows the worker to be open, respectful and curious, thus avoiding a prescriptive or dogmatic approach.

Furthermore, Rapp (2006) proposes six 'recovery principles' these being:

1. *People with psychiatric disabilities can recover, reclaim and transform their lives.*
2. *The focus is on individual strengths rather than deficits.*
3. *The community is viewed as an oasis of resources.*
4. *The client is the director of the helping process.*
5. *The case manager-client relationship is primary and essential.*
6. *The primary setting for the work is the community*

I have received therapy in the past, following traumatic events, which was very helpful and relevant. It can, however, be quite distressing and destructive. I found trying to find a specific cause difficult and, when I looked back at my childhood, saw it as a potential opportunity to blame others for consequences that were out of their and, more importantly, my control.

Looking at what I did and learning from it are very important and this is how potential problems can be worked around in the future. The Scottish Recovery Network, as a good example, acknowledges the importance of traditional therapies too but, in addition, identifies how we can also look forward to better outcomes:

"Traditionally therapy has often been seen as having something to do with 'getting to the root' of problems, expending great effort looking back to the past and trying to analyse the origins of the mental distress or other presenting problems. Whilst a strengths based, solution focused approach does not consider this to necessarily be unhelpful, it does not regard it as the main focus of the process. There is rather more of a future oriented emphasis involving trying to elicit the service user's sense of a 'preferred future'. This can involve the use of various 'what if' questions designed to rekindle a sense within the service user of having permission to dream of an attractive inspiring future. To help this the worker will try to enlist the internal motivations within the person. 'If all the problems that brought you here today just disappeared what would you be doing differently?' 'Where would you be?' 'What would you be doing?' 'How will that be better?'"

If we are looking into the future to see a 'preferred' future, then goal-setting can be a powerful way of capturing things which we would desire to happen in a specific way and time period. We can analyse the past and pick fault with whoever we choose. I have been incredibly guilty of this but the recovery model shows us that we can choose a better path. What good did it do me to torture myself with such destructiveness? Each experience teaches us something new; we have gained, not lost! We can look back also and realise that it was not all bad; and we can build on the times when things went well and learn from any experiences that may not have turned out the way we envisaged. Again, the Scottish Recovery Network provides useful guidance on this:

"Flowing from the self-assessment the service user will then be encouraged to set their own SMART objectives (Specific Measurable Achievable Relevant and Time limited). Negotiating small measurable goals allows for early success to take place and this helps foster motivation toward the next small goal. Having set the goal for themselves the person can see the purpose and meaning of the objective and how it fits with the vision of their preferred future. Small goals are much better than big goals; small goals can create feelings of success and efficacy whereas big goals feel too difficult.

"These goals will be regularly jointly reviewed and serve to help both worker and service user to jointly notice areas of progress and areas of 'stuckness' and to adjust the action plan accordingly. This also allows the service user to identify if appropriate an exit strategy from the support should they feel that they have achieved all the objectives they wanted in collaboration with the service provider. Again this helps maintain a better balance of power and helps prevent creating a dependency."

What Are the Challenges Faced by Clinicians with Recovery Initiatives?

One prime concern that faces many workers is that around patients adopting recovery approaches. Many may show resistance or reluctance, causing more work and pressure for those supporting them. Overseeing one's own decisions may seem very scary for many, or there may be third-party control issues. Changing from having decisions made for you to being in control and more autonomous about decision-making is a huge step. I remember that moving into work from social security benefits was incredibly daunting; yet I also know how hard it was, once being settled, to then to have to leave a job which had formerly been suitable but now no longer was. My view of recovery is about finding things which work and avoiding things which do not. That said, we all have hopes and aspirations – and I do too. Recovery workers are there not only to help patients take more autonomy but also to support clinicians in helping patients make this transitional change. The Nursing In Practice webpage highlights these issues:

"A commonly reported challenge of this approach is the conscious effort needed to consider and engage with patient decisions – particularly when they conflict with the ideas and priorities advocated by working in the medical model framework. In re-establishing control, autonomy and individuality, patient decisions may resist or defy or be incompatible with the risk-averse healthcare culture that has developed within the UK.[17,18]

"Engaging and working with patient choices that seem risky will become an additional source of stress for

healthcare professionals. Nevertheless, for the benefits of this approach to be realised, recovery-orientated practice emphasises building and strengthening patients' positive attributes, positive coping mechanisms and celebrating autonomy.[19]

"Time investment is another challenge presented by this approach because total patient involvement and their pace of change may not coincide with the efficiency pace and time allowances allocated by health practitioners. However, commitment to collaborative working at the patient's pace ensures not only concordance with care interventions but enhances the potential for sustainability.[19] For the practitioner in both instances, using peer support strategies or mechanisms such as case conferences, multi-professionals' meetings and clinical supervision can act as useful forums for gaining support when working with the demands of such challenges.[20]

"Applying the recovery approach to care facilitates and potentiates the individual's prospects for living a meaningful life while adapting and coming to terms with the effects and impact of illness on their mental and physical wellbeing.

"The fundamental skills required to engage in this approach to care are those of effective non-judgmental communication and active listening skills. These, in conjunction with building therapeutic relationships, are deemed key.

"Such skills are already core to effective practice, but embracing this approach will require the progression from total observance and reliance on the traditional medical model of care, where health professionals are deemed the

expert, to a less well-defined role where professionals facilitate and create opportunities for patients to regain autonomy, their own voice and – most importantly – belief in their own ability to direct the transformational processes needed to optimise and adapt to living with their issues."

In more spiritual terms, the above extract emphasises the recovery model's importance in a variety of health and social care settings: in in-patient settings, the community, work and with other agencies such as the Police. The recovery model is not just about one strand but encompasses the way in which a multitude of sectors of the population work and operate.

Conclusion – Wider Benefits of the Recovery Model

Writing this book does, indeed, fill me with hope, particularly when I look at the question of how I have survived all my 'failed' experiences until today! The work-related stress, triggering lack of sleep, mood disturbance and stress from traditional work-related procedures that added negatively to my state of mind – never mind all the battered confidence and having been sectioned at the age of 20 and turbulent times at university – I realise now the importance of continuing to persist in finding some useful employment and I hope, too, that those who are reading this book also recognise the importance of all their experiences. I guess I've never stopped recognising that recovery is a real possibility; I guess that is my strength. I have found a good, straightforward job working as a Sales Consultant for the New Build Sector.

I have found outlets that help me relax, such as acupuncture, holistic therapy and a work/life balance that is sustainable and supports my mental health. For a long time, life wasn't like this; it was tricky and it still has times when things are challenging. I have had at my disposal a loving family who picked up the pieces when I was very poorly in hospital in the year 2000. I have had opportunities that a lot of mental health sufferers have not been able to have which, in many respects, is what has made me want to write about how the help I have had could be so beneficial for others. Many, however, have not had this support and they slip through the net. Some of the approaches that I have detailed, though, may catch those who persistently need help so that they can lead better lives and are therefore able to make better choices. Moreover, I have also covered material that would, as with patients, benefit health professionals too in their own recovery.

I have tried to show at the same time as giving a self-analysis, all the different approaches that the recovery model highlights and how each part can add such tremendous value to our society. Education and training are, in my eyes, at the forefront of ways in which, as has been shown in various Trusts, we can tackle issues such as rising re-admissions, thereby reducing staff sickness absence as well as equipping the mentally disadvantaged with temporary housing to enable them to move forwards, not backwards. Creating a culture based on strengths rather than weaknesses is such a practice that can be adopted not just in a patient/care coordinator role but with the staff themselves, showing support for their needs and identifying tools that can act quickly as a buffer to prevent further negative repercussions. Furthermore, I have given examples of NHS services that have benefited from peer support, showing how those with lived experiences can have a marked impact on the lives of those living with conditions such as eating disorders or drugs and alcohol concerns – these peer support workers show how recovery is a 'bottom-up' approach and the patient is in control of his or her own recovery.

The recovery model is prevalent and available to be practiced in all the areas I have discussed as well as others and there is much potential for considerable growth. For example, I have shown how providing recovery classes could help in ways that are beneficial for patients from things like goal-setting and providing hope to wider, longer term issues such as reducing crime and drug abuse. I have also demonstrated how recovery strategies are interwoven between services, agencies and population groups: employing a strategy in one service can positively impact another service or agency, such as in the work the Police do and in the way staff can benefit from peer support. I have also provided financial evidence to highlight how recovery strategies can really impact NHS budgets positively, showing that the recovery model holds so much intrinsic value that can aid our social and economic development.

References

Anfossi, A (2017), The Current State of Recovery Colleges in the UK, Nottingham: ImROC

Cambridgeshire and Peterborough NHS Foundation Trust (2020), https://www.cpft.nhs.uk/about-us/recovery-college-east.htm

Camden and Islington NHS Foundation Trust (2020), Tile House | Camden and Islington NHS Foundation Trust (candi.nhs.uk)

Coutinho, J, Taking Back Control, London: South West London and St George's Mental Health NHS Trust

Derbyshire Healthcare NHS Foundation Trust (2020), Real life stories::Derbyshire Healthcare NHS Foundation Trust (derbyshirehealthcareft.nhs.uk)

Leeds Recovery College (2020), https://www.leedsandyorkpft.nhs.uk/advice-support/leeds-recovery-college/

Lincolnshire Partnership NHS Foundation Trust (2020), https://www.lpft.nhs.uk/our-services/adults/recovery-college

Maybery, D, and Reupert, A (2018), Families when a parent has a history of mental health problems. From theory to practice (from European Psychiatric/Mental Health Nursing in the 21st century, https://www.researchgate.net/publication/322874181_A_Family-

McCormack, J (2007), Recovery and Strengths Based Practice. SRN Discussion Paper Series. Report No.6, Glasgow: Recovery Network

Miller, Eula, Dr (2017), Clinical: The Recovery approach to life changing conditions, Cogora 26/11/20, https://www.nursinginpractice.com/latest-news/clinical-the-recovery-approach-to-life- changing-conditions/

Merseycare NHS Foundation Trust (2020), No Force First, Mersey Care NHS Foundation Trust – No Force First

NHS England (2020), https://www.england.nhs.uk/mental-health/perinatal/

Perkins, R, Meddings, S, Williams, S, Repper, J, with contributions from Jane Rennison, Joanne Summer, Sharon Gilfoyle and Toni King (2018), Recovery Colleges 10 years on, Nottingham: ImROC

Rinaldi, M, and Wybourn, S (2010), (2011), A Pilot of a Recovery College in the London Boroughs of Merton and Sutton, London: South West London and St George's Mental Health NHS Trust

Slade, M, McDaid, D, Shepherd, G, Williams, and Repper, J (2017), Recovery: The Business Case, Nottingham: ImROC